LOW HISTAMINE COOKBOOK

Discover 1000 Days of Delicious Low-Histamine Recipes for a Healthy Diet, Intolerance Relief, and a Nourishing Food List!

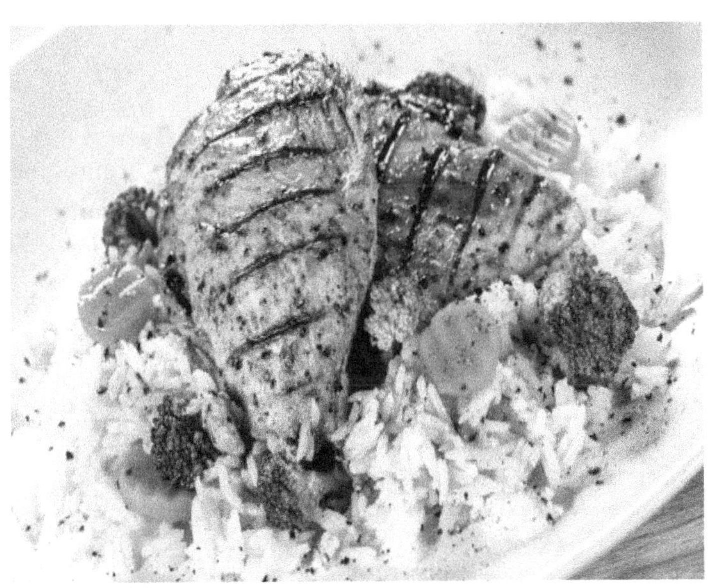

AVELINE WINTER

TABLE OF CONTENT

INTRODUCTION

Have you ever wondered why something as innocent as eating can feel like navigating a culinary minefield? Well, buckle up because Aveline Winter has swooped in with the ultimate solution in her "Low Histamine Cookbook."

Now, let me hit you with a question that might hit close to home: Ever felt like your own body was throwing a food rebellion, leaving you in a constant battle with discomfort and confusion?

Histamine intolerance – it's like your gut decided to play the pickiest food critic ever, and certain ingredients are just not on the guest list. But fear not, because Aveline knows the struggle, and she's got your back.

This cookbook isn't just a collection of recipes; it's your ally in the war against histamine-induced woes. Aveline's carefully chosen meals aren't just about what you can't eat – they're a declaration of what you can. We're talking about detailed ingredients, step-by-step preparation methods, serving sizes that make sense, and nutritional info that's actually useful.

Aveline has cracked the code for ingredient substitutes, ensuring this cookbook is your one-stop-shop, no matter your dietary needs. Miss out on this, and you might as well be turning away from a feast of flavors specifically designed to make histamine intolerance a thing of the past.

If you stop reading now, you're basically telling your taste buds to miss out on a revolutionary journey. This isn't just about cooking; it's about taking back the joy of eating. Imagine meals where you don't have to second-guess every bite. "Low Histamine Cookbook" is not just a book; it's your ticket to a life where food is not the enemy but your partner in crime for a tastier, healthier you.

Ready for the histamine-free revolution? Trust me; you don't want to miss this flavor-packed adventure. Grab a seat at the table, and let's rewrite the rules of your culinary journey!

HOW TO USE THIS COOKBOOK

1. Understand Individual Differences:

- Recognize that everyone's tolerance to histamine varies. Pay attention to your body's reactions and adjust.

2. Thoroughly Review Ingredients:

- Carefully read through each recipe's ingredient list. Take note of any items you know may trigger reactions or that you're sensitive to.

3. Detailed Ingredients and Preparations:

- The cookbook provides detailed lists of ingredients and step-by-step preparation methods for each recipe. Follow them closely to ensure a low histamine outcome.

4. Serving Size Awareness:

- Pay attention to the suggested serving sizes. Adjust portion sizes based on your tolerance levels and individual dietary requirements.

5. Nutritional Information Guidance:

- Check the nutritional information provided for each recipe. This can help you track your intake and ensure it aligns with your dietary goals.

6. Ingredient Substitutes for Flexibility:
- The cookbook includes substitute options to accommodate various dietary needs. Feel free to swap ingredients to suit your preferences or if you have specific allergies.

7. Personalization is Key:
- Understand that the cookbook serves as a guide, but it's crucial to personalize the recipes to fit your unique needs. Modify ingredients or quantities based on your sensitivities.

8. Consult with a Professional:
- If you have severe histamine intolerance or other dietary restrictions, consider consulting with a healthcare professional or nutritionist for personalized advice.

9. Experiment Gradually:
- Introduce new recipes gradually to observe how your body responds. This will help you identify any specific triggers and make informed choices about your meals.

10. Stay Informed and Listen to Your Body:
- Stay informed about histamine-rich foods and how they may impact you. Listen to your body's reaction and adjust your diet accordingly.

Remember, this cookbook is a valuable tool, but your body's response is unique. Use it as a starting point and adapt the recipes to create meals that suit your individual dietary needs and preferences.

CHAPTER 1: FRESH START DELIGHTS

Recipe 1. Zesty Quinoa Salad Burst

Ingredients:

- 1 cup quinoa
- 2 cups water
- 1 cucumber, diced
- 1/2 red bell pepper, diced
- 1/4 cup finely chopped red onion
- 1/4 cup fresh parsley, chopped
- 1/4 cup fresh mint, chopped
- 1/3 cup crumbled feta cheese
- 1/4 cup extra-virgin olive oil
- 2 tablespoons lemon juice
- 1 teaspoon Dijon mustard
- Salt and pepper to taste

Instructions:

1. Rinse the quinoa under cold water. Combine quinoa and water in a medium saucepan . Bring to a boil, then reduce heat, cover, and simmer for 15 minutes or until quinoa is cooked and water is absorbed. Fluff quinoa with a fork and set aside to cool.

2. In a large mixing bowl, combine the cooked quinoa, diced cucumber, diced red bell pepper, chopped red onion, parsley, mint, and crumbled feta cheese.

3. In a small bowl, whisk together olive oil, lemon juice, Dijon mustard, salt, and pepper.

4. Pour the dressing over the quinoa mixture and toss everything until well combined.

5. Chill the salad in the refrigerator for at least 30 minutes before serving to enhance the flavors.

Serving Size:
4 servings

Nutritional Information (per serving):
- Calories: 320
- Protein: 9g
- Fat: 18g
- Carbohydrates: 34g
- Fiber: 5g
- Sugar: 1g

Ingredient Substitutes:
- Quinoa: Replace with cooked brown rice or millet for variety.
- Cucumber: Use zucchini or radishes for a different crunch.
- Red bell pepper: Opt for yellow or orange bell peppers.
- Feta cheese: Choose a lactose-free or goat cheese option.
- Olive oil: Replace with avocado oil or flaxseed oil.
- Lemon juice: Try apple cider vinegar or white wine vinegar.
- Dijon mustard: Use whole grain mustard or omit for a simpler flavor.

Recipe 2. Citrus Infused Grilled Chicken

Ingredients:
- 4 boneless, skinless chicken breasts
- 1/4 cup olive oil
- 2 tablespoons fresh orange juice
- 2 tablespoons fresh lemon juice
- 2 teaspoons honey
- 2 cloves garlic, minced
- 1 teaspoon dried oregano
- 1 teaspoon smoked paprika
- Salt and pepper to taste
- Fresh parsley for garnish

Instructions:
1. In a small bowl, whisk together olive oil, fresh orange juice, fresh lemon juice, honey, minced garlic, dried oregano, smoked paprika, salt, and pepper to create the marinade.
2. Place the chicken breasts in a shallow dish or a zip-top bag and pour half of the marinade over them. Ensure the chicken is well-coated. Reserve the remaining marinade for basting later.
3. Marinate the chicken in the refrigerator for at least 30 minutes, or for a more intense flavor, marinate for up to 4 hours.
4. Preheat the grill to medium-high heat.
5. Remove the chicken from the refrigerator and let it come to room temperature for about 10 minutes.

6. Grill the chicken breasts for 6-8 minutes per side or until the internal temperature reaches 165°F (74°C), basting with the reserved marinade during grilling.
7. Once cooked, remove the chicken from the grill and let it rest for a few minutes.
8. Garnish the grilled chicken with fresh parsley and serve.

Serving Size: 4 servings
Nutritional Information (per serving):
- Calories: 280
- Protein: 28g
- Fat: 15g
- Carbohydrates: 5g
- Fiber: 0.5g
- Sugar: 4g

Ingredient Substitutes:
- Olive oil: Substitute with avocado oil or melted coconut oil.
- Honey: Use maple syrup or agave nectar for a vegan option.
- Dried oregano: Fresh oregano can be used if available.
- Smoked paprika: Regular paprika can be used for a milder flavor.
- Fresh orange and lemon juice: Ensure they are freshly squeezed for optimal flavor.

Note: For those avoiding citrus, consider marinating the chicken in a blend of herbs, garlic, and a suitable acid substitute like vinegar or apple cider.

Recipe 3. Avocado Cucumber Rolls

Ingredients:

- 2 large ripe avocados
- 1 cucumber
- 1 cup cooked quinoa
- 2 tablespoons rice vinegar
- 1 tablespoon sesame oil
- 1 teaspoon soy sauce or tamari for gluten-free
- 1 teaspoon maple syrup or agave nectar
- 1/2 teaspoon black sesame seeds (optional)
- 4 nori sheets

Instructions:

1. In a bowl, mix the cooked quinoa with rice vinegar, sesame oil, soy sauce, and agave nectar. Set aside.
2. Peel the cucumber and slice it into thin strips or use a mandoline for even thickness.
3. Cut the avocados in half, remove the pit, and slice each half into thin strips.
4. Place a nori sheet on a bamboo sushi rolling mat.
5. Wet your hands to prevent sticking and spread about 1/4 cup of the quinoa mixture evenly over the nori sheet, leaving a small border at the top.
6. Arrange cucumber strips and avocado slices along the lower edge of the quinoa.
7. Carefully lift the edge of the nori closest to you, using the rolling mat to guide the ingredients into a tight roll.
8. Wet the top border of the nori sheet with a bit of water to seal the roll.

9. Repeat the process for the remaining nori sheets.

10. Use a sharp knife to slice each roll into bite-sized pieces.

11. Sprinkle with black sesame seeds if desired.

Serving Size: 4 servings

Nutritional Information (per serving):

- Calories: 220

- Protein: 4g

- Fat: 12g

- Carbohydrates: 27g

- Fiber: 6g

- Sugar: 2g

Ingredient Substitutes:

- Quinoa: Replace with cauliflower rice for a lower-carb option.

- Rice vinegar: White wine vinegar or apple cider vinegar can be used.

- Sesame oil: Substitute with avocado oil or a light-flavored oil.

- Soy sauce: Use tamari for a gluten-free alternative or coconut aminos for a soy-free option.

- Agave nectar: Maple syrup, honey, or another liquid sweetener can be used.

- Black sesame seeds: White sesame seeds or chia seeds can be used for a different texture.

Note: These rolls are versatile, and you can customize the filling according to your taste, incorporating ingredients like julienned carrots, bell peppers, or radishes.

Recipe 4. Mango Tango Shrimp Skewers

Ingredients:

- 1 pound of peeled and deveined large shrimp
- 2 ripe mangoes, peeled and cubed
- 1 red bell pepper (cut into chunks)
- 1 red onion, cut into chunks
- 2 tablespoons olive oil
- 2 tablespoons lime juice
- 1 teaspoon chili powder
- 1 teaspoon cumin
- 1/2 teaspoon smoked paprika
- Salt and pepper to taste
- Wooden skewers, soaked in water for about 30 minutes

Instructions:

1. In a bowl, whisk together olive oil, lime juice, chili powder, cumin, smoked paprika, salt, and pepper to create the marinade.

2. Thread shrimp, mango cubes, red bell pepper chunks, and red onion chunks onto the soaked wooden skewers, alternating ingredients.

3. Place the skewers in a shallow dish and brush them generously with the marinade. Let them marinate for at least 15-30 minutes.

4. Preheat the grill pan to medium-high heat.

5. Grill the shrimp skewers for 2-3 minutes per side or until the shrimp are opaque and the vegetables are tender.

6. Brush the skewers with any remaining marinade during grilling for added flavor.

7. Once cooked, remove the skewers from the grill and serve immediately.

Serving Size: 4 servings
Nutritional Information (per serving):
- Calories: 280
- Protein: 22g
- Fat: 10g
- Carbohydrates: 30g
- Fiber: 4g
- Sugar: 22g

Ingredient Substitutes:
- Shrimp: Replace with chicken or tofu for a different protein source.
- Mango: Substitute with pineapple or peach for a sweet and tangy flavor.
- Red bell pepper: Yellow or orange bell peppers can be used for variety.
- Olive oil: Replace with avocado oil or melted coconut oil.
- Lime juice: Lemon juice can be used as a substitute.
- Chili powder: Use paprika for a milder flavor.
- Cumin: Ground coriander or curry powder can be used for a different spice profile.

Note: These skewers can be served with a side of quinoa or a bed of greens for a complete and balanced meal.

Recipe 5. Refreshing Watermelon Gazpacho

Ingredients:

- 4 cups seedless watermelon, diced
- 1 cucumber, peeled and diced
- 1 red bell pepper, diced
- 1/2 red onion, finely chopped
- 2 tablespoons fresh lime juice
- 2 tablespoons olive oil
- 2 tablespoons fresh cilantro, chopped
- 1 teaspoon cumin
- Salt and pepper to taste
- Optional: Jalapeño slices for spice
- Optional: Crumbled feta cheese for garnish

Instructions:

1. In a blender, combine 3 cups of diced watermelon, cucumber, red bell pepper, red onion, fresh lime juice, olive oil, cilantro, and cumin.
2. Blend until smooth and well combined.
3. Season the mixture with salt and pepper for added taste. Adjust the seasoning as needed.
4. Transfer the mixture to a large bowl and stir in the remaining 1 cup of diced watermelon for added texture.
5. Optional: Add jalapeño slices for a spicy kick.
6. Refrigerate the gazpacho for at least 1-2 hours to allow the flavors to meld.
7. Before serving, stir the gazpacho and adjust the seasoning if necessary.

8. Serve the watermelon gazpacho chilled, garnished with optional crumbled feta cheese.

Serving Size: 4 servings

Nutritional Information (per serving):
- Calories: 120
- Protein: 2g
- Fat: 7g
- Carbohydrates: 14g
- Fiber: 2g
- Sugar: 9g

Ingredient Substitutes:
- Cucumber: Use zucchini or celery for a similar crisp texture.
- Red bell pepper: Yellow or orange bell peppers can be used for variety.
- Olive oil: Replace with avocado oil or a light-flavored oil.
- Cilantro: Fresh mint or parsley can be used as alternatives.
- Jalapeño: Adjust the level of spice by adding or omitting this ingredient.
- Feta cheese: Omit for a dairy-free option or replace with crumbled goat cheese.

Note: This watermelon gazpacho is a light and refreshing cold soup, perfect for hot days.

CHAPTER 2: HERB HAVEN CREATIONS

Recipe 6. Basil Pesto Zoodle Bowl

Ingredients:
- 4 medium zucchinis, spiralized into zoodles
- 1 cup cucumber, julienned
- 1/2 cup of pitted and sliced Kalamata olives
- 1/4 cup pine nuts, toasted
- 1/2 cup fresh basil leaves
- 1/4 cup nutritional yeast
- 1/3 cup extra-virgin olive oil
- 2 cloves garlic, minced
- Salt and pepper to taste

Instructions:
1. In a blender or food processor, combine basil, nutritional yeast, garlic, and pine nuts. Pulse until coarsely chopped.
2. With the blender or food processor running, slowly stream in the olive oil until the pesto reaches a smooth consistency.
3. In a large bowl, toss the zoodles with julienne cucumber, Kalamata olives, and the prepared pesto.
4. Season with salt and pepper to taste.
5. Serve the zoodle bowl chilled, optionally topped with extra pine nuts and fresh basil.

Serving Size:
4 servings

Nutritional Information (per serving):
- Calories: 280
- Protein: 5g
- Fat: 22g
- Carbohydrates: 14g
- Fiber: 4g
- Sugar: 5g

Ingredient Substitutes:
- Zucchini: Substitute with spiralized cucumber or daikon radish for variety.
- Pine nuts: Use sunflower seeds or pepitas as a nut alternative.
- Nutritional yeast: Omit for a different flavor or add a small amount of goat cheese for some creaminess.
- Olive oil: Avocado oil or hemp oil can be used.
- Cucumber: Radishes or jicama can be used for a similar crisp texture.

Recipe 7. Rosemary Roasted Salmon

Ingredients:
- 4 salmon filets
- 2 tablespoons olive oil
- 2 tablespoons fresh rosemary, chopped
- 2 cloves garlic, minced
- 1 lemon, sliced
- Salt and pepper to taste

Instructions:
1. Preheat the oven to 400°F (200°C).
2. On a baking sheet, place salmon filets lined with parchment paper.
3. In a small bowl, mix olive oil, chopped rosemary, minced garlic, salt, and pepper.
4. Brush the rosemary mixture over the salmon filets.
5. Top each filet with lemon slices.
6. Bake in the preheated oven for 12-15 minutes or until the salmon is cooked through and flakes easily with a fork.
7. Serve the rosemary roasted salmon with a side of steamed green beans or your choice of low histamine vegetables.

Serving Size:
4 servings

Nutritional Information (per serving):
- Calories: 300
- Protein: 25g
- Fat: 20g
- Carbohydrates: 2g
- Fiber: 0.5g
- Sugar: 0.5g

Ingredient Substitutes:
- Salmon: Substitute with another low histamine fish such as trout or cod.
- Rosemary: Thyme or oregano can be used for a different herb flavor.
- Olive oil: Avocado oil or melted ghee can be alternatives.
- Lemon: Use lime or orange slices for a citrusy twist.

Recipe 8. Minty Lemon Chicken Lettuce Wraps

Ingredients:
- 1 pound ground chicken
- 1 tablespoon olive oil
- 2 tablespoons fresh mint, finely chopped
- 1 lemon, juiced and zested
- 2 cloves garlic, minced
- Salt and pepper to taste
- Iceberg or butter lettuce leaves, for serving
- Radish slices for garnish

Instructions:
1. In a skillet over medium heat, add olive oil and sauté minced garlic until fragrant.
2. Add ground chicken and cook until it's brown, breaking it apart with a spoon.
3. Stir in fresh mint, lemon juice, lemon zest, salt, and pepper. Cook for an additional 2-3 minutes.
4. Spoon the chicken mixture onto individual lettuce leaves.
5. Garnish with radish slices for an extra crunch.
6. Serve the minty lemon chicken lettuce wraps immediately.

Serving Size:
4 servings

Nutritional Information (per serving):
- Calories: 230
- Protein: 20g
- Fat: 15g
- Carbohydrates: 4g
- Fiber: 1g
- Sugar: 1g

Ingredient Substitutes:
- Ground chicken: Substitute with ground turkey or tofu crumbles for a plant-based option.
- Olive oil: Avocado oil or coconut oil can be used.
- Mint: Use fresh basil or cilantro for a different herb flavor.
- Lettuce: Bibb lettuce or Romaine leaves can be used instead of iceberg.
- Radish: Jicama or cucumber slices can be used for a similar crisp texture.

Recipe 9. Dill Infused Cucumber Salad

Ingredients:

- 3 medium cucumbers, thinly sliced
- 1/4 cup fresh dill, chopped
- 1/4 cup red onion, thinly sliced
- 2 tablespoons olive oil
- 2 tablespoons white wine vinegar
- 1 teaspoon Dijon mustard
- Salt and pepper to taste

Instructions:

1. In a large bowl, combine thinly sliced cucumbers, chopped dill, and thinly sliced red onion.

2. In a separate small bowl, whisk together olive oil, white wine vinegar, Dijon mustard, salt, and pepper.

3. Pour the dressing over the cucumber mixture and toss until well mixed.

4. Let the cucumber salad marinate in the refrigerator for about 30 minutes to allow the flavors to meld.

5. Serve the dill-infused cucumber salad chilled, garnished with additional dill if desired.

Serving Size:

4 servings

Nutritional Information (per serving):
- Calories: 90
- Protein: 1g
- Fat: 7g
- Carbohydrates: 8g
- Fiber: 2g
- Sugar: 4g

Ingredient Substitutes:
- Cucumbers: Use English cucumbers or Persian cucumbers for a milder flavor.
- Red onion: Green onions or chives can be used for a different onion flavor.
- Olive oil: Avocado oil or flaxseed oil can be alternatives.
- White wine vinegar: Apple cider vinegar or rice vinegar can be used.
- Dijon mustard: Yellow mustard or grainy mustard for variety.

Recipe 10. Coriander-Crusted Cod Filets

Ingredients:
- 4 cod filets
- 2 tablespoons coriander powder
- 1 tablespoon olive oil
- 1 teaspoon ground cumin
- 1/2 teaspoon ground turmeric
- Salt and pepper to taste
- Lemon wedges for serving

Instructions:
1. Preheat the oven to 400°F (200°C).
2. In a small bowl, mix coriander powder, ground cumin, ground turmeric, salt, and pepper.
3. Pat the cod filets dry and rub the spice mixture evenly on both sides.
4. Heat olive oil in an oven-safe skillet over medium-high heat.
5. Sear the cod filets for 2 minutes on each side to develop a crust.
6. Transfer the skillet to the preheated oven and bake for 8-10 minutes or until the cod is cooked through and flakes easily.
7. Serve the coriander-crusted cod filets with lemon wedges.

Serving Size:
4 servings

Nutritional Information (per serving):
- Calories: 180
- Protein: 22g
- Fat: 8g
- Carbohydrates: 2g
- Fiber: 1g
- Sugar: 0g

Ingredient Substitutes:
- Cod filets: Substitute with another low histamine fish like haddock or trout.
- Coriander powder: Use ground cumin or fennel for a different spice profile.
- Olive oil: Avocado oil or melted ghee can be alternatives.
- Ground turmeric: Ground ginger or paprika for a mild spice.

CHAPTER 3: RAINBOW HARMONY FEAST

Recipe 11. Colorful Bell Pepper Stir-Fry

Ingredients:

- 2 red bell peppers, sliced
- 2 yellow bell peppers, sliced
- 2 green bell peppers, sliced
- 1 medium carrot, julienned
- 1 zucchini, sliced
- 2 tablespoons olive oil
- 2 cloves garlic, minced
- 1 teaspoon fresh ginger, grated
- 1 tablespoon tamari (gluten-free soy sauce)
- 1 teaspoon sesame oil
- Sesame seeds for garnish
- Fresh cilantro for garnish

Instructions:

1. Heat olive oil over medium-high heat in a large skillet or wok.

2. Add minced garlic and grated ginger, sauté for 1-2 minutes until fragrant.

3. Add sliced bell peppers, julienned carrot, and sliced zucchini to the skillet. Stir-fry for 4-5 minutes until vegetables are tender yet crisp.

4. Drizzle tamari and sesame oil over the vegetables, toss to combine.

5. Continue to stir-fry for an additional 2-3 minutes until the flavors meld.

6. Garnish the colorful bell pepper stir-fry with sesame seeds and fresh cilantro.

7. Serve immediately on its own or over low histamine rice alternatives like quinoa or millet.

Serving Size:
4 servings

Nutritional Information (per serving):
- Calories: 120
- Protein: 2g
- Fat: 7g
- Carbohydrates: 14g
- Fiber: 4g
- Sugar: 7g

Ingredient Substitutes:
- Bell peppers: Substitute with low histamine vegetables like jicama, bok choy, or cucumber.
- Tamari: Use coconut aminos for a soy-free option.
- Olive oil: Avocado oil or coconut oil can be used.
- Sesame oil: Substitute with flaxseed oil for a different nutty flavor.

Recipe 12. Turmeric Spiced Cauliflower Rice

Ingredients:

- 1 medium-sized cauliflower, grated (or 4 cups store-bought cauliflower rice)
- 2 tablespoons olive oil
- 1 teaspoon turmeric powder
- 1/2 teaspoon ground cumin
- 1/2 teaspoon ground coriander
- Salt and pepper to taste
- Fresh parsley for garnish

Instructions:

1. Heat olive oil over medium heat, in a large skillet.
2. Add grated cauliflower to the skillet, stirring occasionally for 3-4 minutes until it starts to soften.
3. Sprinkle turmeric powder, ground cumin, and ground coriander over the cauliflower. Mix well to distribute the spices evenly.
4. Continue cooking for an additional 5-7 minutes until the cauliflower rice is cooked through.
5. Season with salt and pepper to taste, adjusting as needed.
6. Garnish with fresh parsley before serving.
7. Serve the turmeric spiced cauliflower rice as a base for various dishes.

Serving Size:

4 servings

Nutritional Information (per serving):
- Calories: 80
- Protein: 3g
- Fat: 6g
- Carbohydrates: 6g
- Fiber: 3g
- Sugar: 2g

Ingredient Substitutes:
- Cauliflower: Use broccoli or jicama as a low histamine alternative.
- Turmeric powder: Use ginger powder for a slightly different flavor.
- Olive oil: Avocado oil or ghee can be used.

Recipe 13. Broccoli and Carrot Ribbon Salad

Ingredients:
- 2 cups broccoli florets
- 2 large carrots, peeled into ribbons
- 1/4 cup sunflower seeds, toasted
- 2 tablespoons olive oil
- 1 tablespoon apple cider vinegar
- 1 teaspoon honey (optional)
- 1 teaspoon Dijon mustard
- Salt and pepper to taste
- Fresh parsley for garnish

Instructions:
1. Steam the broccoli florets for 2-3 minutes until they are slightly tender but still crisp.
2. Using a vegetable peeler, peel the carrots into ribbons.
3. In a large bowl, combine the broccoli florets, carrot ribbons, and toasted sunflower seeds.
4. In a small bowl, whisk together olive oil, apple cider vinegar, honey (if using), Dijon mustard, salt, and pepper.
5. Pour the dressing over the vegetables and toss until well mixed.
6. Garnish the broccoli and carrot ribbon salad with fresh parsley.
7. Refrigerate for later use or serve immediately.

Serving Size:
4 servings

Nutritional Information (per serving):
- Calories: 120
- Protein: 3g
- Fat: 9g
- Carbohydrates: 10g
- Fiber: 4g
- Sugar: 5g

Ingredient Substitutes:
- Broccoli: Use cauliflower or asparagus for a different texture.
- Sunflower seeds: Substitute with pumpkin seeds or chopped almonds.
- Olive oil: Avocado oil or flaxseed oil can be used.
- Apple cider vinegar: White wine vinegar or rice vinegar for a milder flavor.
- Honey: Replace with maple syrup or agave nectar for a vegan option.

Recipe 14. Purple Potato Mash Delight

Ingredients:
- 4 medium-sized purple potatoes, peeled and diced
- 2 tablespoons olive oil
- 1/4 cup unsweetened almond milk (or any low histamine milk alternative)
- 1 teaspoon garlic powder
- Salt and pepper to taste
- Chives for garnish

Instructions:
1. Place the diced purple potatoes in a pot and cover with water. Bring to a boil and simmer until the potatoes are fork-tender, at least 15 minutes.
2. Drain the potatoes and put them in the pot.
3. Mash the potatoes using a potato masher or fork until smooth.
4. Add olive oil, almond milk, garlic powder, salt, and pepper to the mashed potatoes. Mix until well combined.
5. Adjust the seasoning to taste.
6. Garnish the purple potato mash with chopped chives.
7. Serve the mash as a delightful and colorful side dish.

Serving Size:
4 servings

Nutritional Information (per serving):
- Calories: 180
- Protein: 3g
- Fat: 7g
- Carbohydrates: 27g
- Fiber: 4g
- Sugar: 2g

Ingredient Substitutes:
- Purple potatoes: Use sweet potatoes or regular potatoes for a different color and flavor.
- Olive oil: Avocado oil or coconut oil can be used.
- Almond milk: Substitute with any low histamine milk alternative like coconut milk or rice milk.

Recipe 15. Green Bean Almondine Bliss

Ingredients:
- 1 pound green beans, ends trimmed
- 2 tablespoons olive oil
- 1/3 cup sliced almonds, toasted
- 2 tablespoons fresh lemon juice
- 1 teaspoon lemon zest
- 2 cloves garlic, minced
- Salt and pepper to taste
- Fresh parsley for garnish

Instructions:
1. Blanch the green beans in boiling water for 2-3 minutes until they are bright green and slightly tender. Transfer them immediately to an ice water bath to stop the cooking process. Drain and set aside.
2. In a large skillet, heat olive oil over medium heat.
3. Add minced garlic and sauté for 1-2 minutes until fragrant.
4. Add the blanched green beans to the skillet, tossing to coat them in the garlic-infused oil.
5. Stir in toasted sliced almonds and continue to sauté for an additional 2-3 minutes until the green beans are heated through.
6. Drizzle fresh lemon juice over the green beans and sprinkle with lemon zest.
7. Season with salt and pepper to taste. Toss everything together.

8. Garnish the green bean almondine with fresh parsley before serving.

Serving Size:
4 servings

Nutritional Information (per serving):
- Calories: 120
- Protein: 3g
- Fat: 9g
- Carbohydrates: 9g
- Fiber: 4g
- Sugar: 3g

Ingredient Substitutes:
- Green beans: Use asparagus or snap peas for a different twist.
- Sliced almonds: Substitute with pine nuts or chopped hazelnuts.
- Olive oil: Avocado oil or ghee can be alternatives.
- Lemon: Use lime for a citrusy variation.

CHAPTER 4: MEDITERRANEAN MAGIC EXTRAVAGANZA

Recipe 16. Greek Salad Quinoa Bowl

Ingredients:

- 1 cup quinoa, rinsed and cooked
- 1 cup cucumber, diced
- 1 cup cherry tomatoes, halved
- 1/2 cup of pitted and sliced Kalamata olives
- 1/2 cup red bell pepper, diced
- 1/4 cup red onion, finely chopped
- 1/3 cup crumbled feta cheese (optional)
- 2 tablespoons extra-virgin olive oil
- 1 tablespoon red wine vinegar
- 1 teaspoon dried oregano
- Salt and pepper to taste
- Fresh parsley for garnish

Instructions:

1. In a large bowl, combine cooked quinoa, diced cucumber, halved cherry tomatoes, sliced Kalamata olives, diced red bell pepper, and finely chopped red onion.
2. Whisk together olive oil, red wine vinegar, dried oregano, salt, and pepper, in a small bowl.
3. Pour the dressing over the quinoa mixture and toss until well combined.
4. If using, sprinkle crumbled feta cheese over the top.
5. Garnish the Greek salad quinoa bowl with fresh parsley.
6. Serve immediately or refrigerate for later use.

Serving Size:
4 servings

Nutritional Information (per serving):
- Calories: 280
- Protein: 8g
- Fat: 14g
- Carbohydrates: 32g
- Fiber: 5g
- Sugar: 3g

Ingredient Substitutes:
- Quinoa: Use cauliflower rice or millet for a different base.
- Feta cheese: Omit for a dairy-free option or substitute with dairy-free feta.
- Red wine vinegar: White wine vinegar or apple cider vinegar can be used.
- Kalamata olives: Use green olives or omit for those sensitive to olives.

Recipe 17. Lemon Dill Baked Tilapia

Ingredients:
- 4 tilapia filets
- 2 tablespoons olive oil
- 2 tablespoons fresh lemon juice
- 1 tablespoon fresh dill, chopped
- 1 teaspoon lemon zest
- 2 cloves garlic, minced
- Salt and pepper to taste
- Lemon slices for garnish

Instructions:
1. Preheat the oven to 375°F (190°C).
2. Place tilapia filets in a baking pan.
3. In a small bowl, whisk together olive oil, fresh lemon juice, chopped dill, lemon zest, minced garlic, salt, and pepper.
4. Pour the lemon dill mixture over the tilapia filets, ensuring they are well-coated.
5. Arrange lemon slices on top of each filet.
6. Bake in the preheated oven for 15-20 minutes or until the tilapia is cooked through and flakes easily.
7. Garnish with additional fresh dill before serving.

Serving Size:
4 servings

Nutritional Information (per serving):
- Calories: 180
- Protein: 25g
- Fat: 8g
- Carbohydrates: 2g
- Fiber: 0.5g
- Sugar: 0.5g

Ingredient Substitutes:
- Tilapia: Substitute with cod, haddock, or another low histamine fish.
- Olive oil: Avocado oil or melted ghee can be alternatives.
- Lemon: Use lime for a slightly different citrus flavor.

Recipe 18. Minty Tzatziki Cucumber Cups

Ingredients:
- 3 medium cucumbers
- 1 cup Greek yogurt or dairy-free alternative
- 1/4 cup fresh mint, finely chopped
- 1 clove garlic, minced
- 1 tablespoon extra-virgin olive oil
- 1 tablespoon lemon juice
- Salt and pepper to taste
- Cherry tomatoes for garnish

Instructions:
1. Peel the cucumbers and cut them into 1-inch thick slices.
2. Use a melon baller or spoon to hollow out the centers of each cucumber slice, creating cups.
3. In a bowl, combine Greek yogurt, finely chopped mint, minced garlic, olive oil, lemon juice, salt, and pepper.
4. Spoon the minty tzatziki mixture into each cucumber cup.
5. Garnish with cherry tomato halves on top.
6. Serve immediately as a refreshing appetizer or snack.

Nutritional Information (per serving):
- Calories: 80
- Protein: 5g
- Fat: 4g
- Carbohydrates: 6g
- Fiber: 1g
- Sugar: 3g

Serving size:
Approximately 12 cucumber cups

Ingredient Substitutes:

- Greek yogurt: Use dairy-free yogurt for a vegan option.
- Fresh mint: Substitute with fresh dill or parsley for a different herb flavor.
- Olive oil: Avocado oil or flaxseed oil can be alternatives.
- Cherry tomatoes: Use diced cucumber or red bell pepper for a different garnish.

Recipe 19 Cucumber Olive Salsa Fiesta

Ingredients:

- 2 medium cucumbers, diced
- 1 cup of pitted and sliced Kalamata olives
- 1/2 red onion, finely chopped
- 1/4 cup fresh cilantro, chopped
- 2 tablespoons extra-virgin olive oil
- 1 tablespoon red wine vinegar
- 1 teaspoon dried oregano
- Salt and pepper to taste
- Jalapeño slices for optional spice

Instructions:

1. In a large bowl, combine diced cucumbers, sliced Kalamata olives, finely chopped red onion, and chopped cilantro.

2. Whisk together olive oil, red wine vinegar, dried oregano, salt, and pepper, in a small bowl.

3. Pour the dressing over the cucumber olive salsa and toss until well combined.

4. Add jalapeño slices if you desire a spicy kick.

5. Refrigerate the salsa for about 30 minutes to allow the flavors to meld.

6. Serve the cucumber olive salsa as a refreshing side dish or on top of grilled fish or chicken.

Nutritional Information (per serving):
- Calories: 120
- Protein: 2g
- Fat: 10g
- Carbohydrates: 7g
- Fiber: 2g
- Sugar: 3g
Sodium: 50mg

Serving size: 4 cups

Ingredient Substitutes:

- Kalamata olives: Use green olives or black olives as an alternative.
- Red wine vinegar: White wine vinegar or apple cider vinegar can be used.
- Fresh cilantro: Substitute with fresh parsley or basil for a different herb flavor.
- Jalapeño slices: Adjust the level of spice based on personal preference.

Recipe 20. Mediterranean Veggie Skewers

Ingredients:
- 1 zucchini, sliced into rounds
- 1 red bell pepper, in chunks
- 1 yellow bell pepper, cut into chunks
- 1 red onion, cut into wedges
- 8 oz mushrooms, cleaned and halved
- 2 tablespoons olive oil
- 2 teaspoons dried oregano
- 1 teaspoon dried thyme
- 1 teaspoon garlic powder
- Salt and pepper to taste
- Wooden skewers, soaked in water for about 30 minutes

Instructions:
1. Preheat the grill or grill pan on medium-high heat.
2. In a large bowl, combine zucchini, red bell pepper, yellow bell pepper, red onion, and mushrooms.
3. In a small bowl, whisk together olive oil, dried oregano, dried thyme, garlic powder, salt, and pepper.
4. Pour the olive oil mixture over the vegetables and toss until evenly coated.
5. Thread the marinated vegetables onto the soaked wooden skewers, alternating the vegetables for a colorful mix.
6. Place the skewers on the preheated grill and cook for about 8-10 minutes, turning occasionally, until the vegetables are tender and slightly charred.

7. Remove the skewers from the grill and let them rest for a few minutes.

Serving Size: 4 skewers

Nutritional Information (per serving):
- Calories: 120
- Fat: 9g
- Carbohydrates: 10g
- Fiber: 4g
- Protein: 3g

Ingredient Substitutes:
- Zucchini: Yellow squash or eggplant
- Red/Yellow Bell Pepper: Green bell pepper or other colorful bell peppers
- Red Onion: White onion or shallots
- Mushrooms: Asparagus or other preferred vegetables
- Olive Oil: Grapeseed oil or avocado oil
- Dried Oregano/Thyme: Fresh herbs if available
- Garlic Powder: Minced garlic cloves

CHAPTER 5: BERRY BLISSFUL TREATS

Recipe 21. Blueberry Walnut Chicken Salad

Ingredients:
- 2 cups cooked chicken breast, shredded
- 1 cup blueberries
- 1/2 cup walnuts, chopped
- 1/2 cup celery, finely diced
- 1/4 cup red onion, finely chopped
- 1/4 cup fresh parsley, chopped
- 1/3 cup mayonnaise (or dairy-free alternative)
- 1 tablespoon Dijon mustard
- 1 tablespoon apple cider vinegar
- Salt and pepper to taste
- Lettuce leaves for serving

Instructions:
1. In a large bowl, combine shredded chicken, blueberries, chopped walnuts, diced celery, chopped red onion, and fresh parsley.
2. In a separate small bowl, whisk together mayonnaise, Dijon mustard, apple cider vinegar, salt, and pepper to create the dressing.
3. Pour the dressing over the chicken mixture and toss until all ingredients are well-coated.
4. Refrigerate the salad for at least 30 minutes to let the flavors meld.

5. Serve the blueberry walnut chicken salad on crisp lettuce leaves.

Serving Size: 4 servings

Nutritional Information (per serving):
- Calories: 320
- Protein: 20g
- Fat: 25g
- Carbohydrates: 10g
- Fiber: 3g
- Sugar: 5g

Ingredient Substitutes:
- Blueberries: Use strawberries or raspberries for a different berry flavor.
- Walnuts: Substitute with almonds, pecans, or sunflower seeds.
- Mayonnaise: Use Greek yogurt or a dairy-free yogurt alternative.
- Dijon mustard: Yellow mustard or grainy mustard can be used.

Recipe 22. Mango Berry Coconut Smoothie

Ingredients:

- 1 cup frozen mango chunks
- 1/2 cup mixed berries such as blueberries, strawberries, or raspberries
- 1/2 cup coconut milk (canned or carton)
- 1/2 cup water or coconut water
- 1 tablespoon chia seeds
- 1 tablespoon shredded coconut (unsweetened)
- 1 teaspoon maple syrup or honey (optional)
- Ice cubes (optional)

Instructions:

1. In a blender, combine frozen mango chunks, mixed berries, coconut milk, water, chia seeds, and shredded coconut.
2. Blend until smooth and creamy. Add more liquid if needed.
3. Taste the smoothie and add honey or maple syrup if additional sweetness is desired.
4. If you prefer a colder smoothie, add ice cubes and blend again.
5. Pour the mango berry coconut smoothie into a glass and garnish with extra shredded coconut if desired.
6. Serve immediately and enjoy the tropical flavors!

Serving Size: 2 servings

Nutritional Information (per serving):
- Calories: 220
- Protein: 3g
- Fat: 12g
- Carbohydrates: 28g
- Fiber: 6g
- Sugar: 18g

Ingredient Substitutes:
- Use any low histamine fruits like peaches or pineapple.
- Substitute coconut milk with almond milk or another low histamine milk alternative.
- Chia seeds and shredded coconut can be omitted if needed.

Recipe 23. Raspberry Chia Seed Pudding

Ingredients:
- 1 cup frozen or fresh raspberries
- 1/4 cup chia seeds
- 1 cup coconut milk (canned or carton)
- 1 tablespoon maple syrup or honey
- 1/2 teaspoon vanilla extract
- Fresh raspberries for garnish

Instructions:

1. In a blender, combine fresh or frozen raspberries, chia seeds, coconut milk, maple syrup (or honey), and vanilla extract.

2. Blend until the mixture is smooth and well combined.

3. Pour the raspberry chia seed mixture into jars or bowls.

4. Cover and refrigerate for at least 4 hours or overnight to allow the chia seeds to absorb the liquid and form a pudding-like consistency.

5. Before serving, give the pudding a good stir to ensure an even texture.

6. Garnish with fresh raspberries before serving.

Serving Size: 2 servings

Nutritional Information (per serving):
- Calories: 220
- Protein: 4g
- Fat: 14g
- Carbohydrates: 22g
- Fiber: 8g
- Sugar: 8g

Ingredient Substitutes:
- Replace raspberries with strawberries or blueberries.
- Use almond milk or another low histamine milk alternative.
- Adjust sweetener based on personal preference or dietary needs.

Recipe 24. Blackberry Mint Sorbet

Ingredients:
- 2 cups blackberries
- 1/4 cup fresh mint leaves
- 1/4 cup honey or agave nectar
- 1 tablespoon fresh lime juice
- 1/2 cup water

Instructions:
1. In a blender, combine blackberries, fresh mint leaves, honey (or agave nectar), fresh lime juice, and water.
2. Blend until smooth.
3. Strain the mixture through a fine mesh sieve to remove seeds and mint leaves.
4. Pour the sorbet base into an ice cream maker and churn according to the manufacturer's instructions.
5. Transfer the churned sorbet to a lidded container and freeze for an additional 2 hours to firm up.
6. Scoop the blackberry mint sorbet into bowls or cones.
7. Garnish with fresh mint leaves before serving.

Nutritional Information (per serving):
- Calories: 120g
- Protein: 1g
- Fat: 0g
- Carbohydrates: 30g
- Fiber: 7g
- Sugar: 23g

Serving size: 4 servings

Ingredient Substitutes:
- Replace blackberries with blueberries or raspberries.
- Adjust sweetener based on personal preference or dietary needs.

Recipe 25. Cherry Almond Yogurt Parfait

Ingredients:

- 1 cup fresh or frozen cherries, pitted and halved
- 1 cup dairy-free yogurt (coconut or almond yogurt)
- 1/4 cup almond slices, toasted
- 2 tablespoons chia seeds
- 1 tablespoon maple syrup or honey
- 1/2 teaspoon almond extract (optional)
- Fresh mint leaves for garnish

Instructions:

1. In a bowl, mix cherries with maple syrup (or honey) and let them sit for a few minutes to release their juices.
2. In a separate bowl, combine dairy-free yogurt with almond extract if using.
3. In serving glasses or bowls, layer the yogurt, followed by the cherry mixture, toasted almond slices, and chia seeds.
4. Repeat the layers until the glasses are filled, ending with a layer of cherries and a sprinkle of almond slices.
5. Garnish with fresh mint leaves.
6. Refrigerate for about 30 minutes to allow the flavors to meld.
7. Serve the cherry almond yogurt parfait chilled.

Serving Size: 2 servings

Nutritional Information (per serving):
- Calories: 250
- Protein: 6g
- Fat: 12g
- Carbohydrates: 32g
- Fiber: 7g
- Sugar: 19g

Ingredient Substitutes:
- Replace cherries with another low histamine fruit like peaches or strawberries.
- Choose any dairy-free yogurt alternative based on preference.
- Adjust sweetener based on personal preference or dietary needs.

CHAPTER 6: LOW HISTAMINE SNACK SENSATIONS

Recipe 26. Crispy Chickpea Crunch

Ingredients:

- 2 cans (15 oz each) of drained and rinsed chickpeas
- 2 tablespoons olive oil
- 1 teaspoon ground cumin
- 1 teaspoon smoked paprika
- 1/2 teaspoon garlic powder
- 1/2 teaspoon onion powder
- 1/2 teaspoon sea salt
- 1/4 teaspoon black pepper
- 1/4 teaspoon cayenne pepper for added heat (optional)

Instructions:

1.Line a baking sheet with parchment paper, then preheat the oven to 400°F (200°C).

2. Pat the chickpeas dry with a paper towel to reduce excess moisture.

3. In a bowl, toss the chickpeas with olive oil, ground cumin, smoked paprika, garlic powder, onion powder, sea salt, black pepper, and cayenne pepper if using.

4. Spread the seasoned chickpeas in a single layer on the prepared baking sheet.

5. Bake in the preheated oven for 30-40 minutes or until the chickpeas are crispy and golden brown, shaking the pan halfway through the cooking time.

6. Remove from the oven and let them cool for a few minutes before serving.

7. Enjoy the crispy chickpea crunch as a snack or sprinkle them over salads for added texture.

Serving size: 2 cups

Nutritional Information (per 1/2 cup serving):
- Calories: 130
- Protein: 5g
- Fat: 6g
- Carbohydrates: 15g
- Fiber: 4g
- Sugar: 3g

Ingredient Substitutes:
- Experiment with different spice combinations like curry powder, turmeric, or cajun seasoning.
- Use avocado oil or coconut oil instead of olive oil.
- Adjust the level of cayenne pepper based on personal spice preference.

Recipe 27. Spiced Pumpkin Seed Mix

Ingredients:
- 1 cup raw pumpkin seeds (pepitas)
- 1 tablespoon olive oil
- 1 teaspoon ground cumin
- 1/2 teaspoon smoked paprika
- 1/2 teaspoon garlic powder
- 1/2 teaspoon onion powder
- 1/2 teaspoon sea salt
- 1/4 teaspoon black pepper
- Pinch of cayenne pepper (optional for added heat)

Instructions:
1. Preheat the oven to 325°F (163°C) then line a baking sheet with parchment paper.
2. In a bowl, toss the raw pumpkin seeds with olive oil, ground cumin, smoked paprika, garlic powder, onion powder, sea salt, black pepper, and cayenne pepper if using.
3. Spread the seasoned pumpkin seeds in a single layer on the prepared baking sheet.
4. Bake in the preheated oven for 15-20 minutes, stirring occasionally, until the pumpkin seeds are golden brown and crispy.
5. Remove from the oven and let them cool completely before serving or storing.
6. Enjoy the spiced pumpkin seed mix as a nutritious snack or add it to salads for extra crunch.

Serving Size: 1 cup

Nutritional Information (per 1/4 cup serving):
- Calories: 100
- Protein: 5g
- Fat: 8g
- Carbohydrates: 3g
- Fiber: 1g
- Sugar: 0g

Ingredient Substitutes:
- Experiment with different spice combinations like chili powder, turmeric, or rosemary.
- Use melted coconut oil or avocado oil instead of olive oil.
- Adjust the level of cayenne pepper based on personal spice preference.

Recipe 28. Cucumber Dill Hummus Cups

Ingredients:
- 2 medium cucumbers
- 1 cup hummus (store-bought or homemade)
- 2 tablespoons fresh dill, chopped
- 1 tablespoon lemon juice
- Salt and pepper to taste
- Cherry tomatoes for garnish (optional)

Instructions:
1. Peel the cucumbers and cut them into 1-inch thick slices.
2. Use a melon baller or spoon to hollow out the centers of each cucumber slice, creating cups.
3. In a bowl, combine hummus, chopped fresh dill, lemon juice, salt, and pepper. Mix well.
4. Spoon the hummus mixture into each cucumber cup.
5. Garnish with cherry tomato halves if desired.
6. Serve the cucumber dill hummus cups as a refreshing appetizer or snack.

Nutritional Information (per serving):
- Calories: 150g
- Protein: 5g
- Fat: 10g
- Carbohydrates: 14g
- Fiber: 4g
- Sugar: 3g

Serving Size: Approximately 12 cucumber cups

Ingredient Substitutes:
- Experiment with different herb combinations like parsley or mint.
- Customize hummus flavors based on personal preference.
- Add diced bell peppers or olives for additional flavor and texture.

Recipe 29. Sliced Apple Almond Butter Bites

Ingredients:
- 2 medium apples, sliced
- 1/2 cup almond butter
- 2 tablespoons chia seeds
- 2 tablespoons unsweetened shredded coconut
- 1 tablespoon honey or maple syrup (optional)
- 1/2 teaspoon cinnamon
- Squeeze of lemon juice

Instructions:
1. Slice the apples into thin rounds then arrange them on a serving plate.
2. In a small bowl, mix almond butter, chia seeds, shredded coconut, honey or maple syrup (if using), and cinnamon.
3. Squeeze a bit of lemon juice over the apple slices to prevent browning.
4. Spread a dollop of the almond butter mixture onto each apple slice.
5. Optional: Drizzle with extra honey or sprinkle additional chia seeds on top.
6. Serve the sliced apple almond butter bites as a delightful and nutritious snack.

Serving Size; 16 almond butter bites

Nutritional Information (per 4 bites):
- Calories: 200
- Protein: 5g
- Fat: 15g
- Carbohydrates: 15g
- Fiber: 5g
- Sugar: 9g

Ingredient Substitutes:
- Use peanut butter or sunflower seed butter as an alternative to almond butter.
- Customize toppings with crushed nuts or seeds for added crunch.
- Adjust sweetness based on personal preference.

Recipe 30. Trail Mix with Walnuts and Dried Cranberries

Ingredients:

- 1 cup walnuts
- 1/2 cup pumpkin seeds (pepitas)
- 1/2 cup sunflower seeds
- 1/2 cup unsweetened dried cranberries
- 1/4 cup unsweetened shredded coconut
- 1/2 teaspoon ground cinnamon
- 1/4 teaspoon sea salt

Instructions:

1. In a dry skillet over medium heat, toast walnuts, pumpkin seeds, and sunflower seeds until they are lightly golden and fragrant. Stir frequently to prevent burning.

2. Allow the toasted nuts and seeds to cool completely.

3. In a bowl, combine toasted walnuts, pumpkin seeds, sunflower seeds, dried cranberries, shredded coconut, ground cinnamon, and sea salt. Toss until well mixed.

4. Transfer the trail mix to an airtight container for storage.

5. Enjoy the trail mix with walnuts and dried cranberries as a convenient and satisfying snack.

Serving Size: 2 cups

Nutritional Information (per 1/4 cup serving):
- Calories: 150
- Protein: 4g
- Fat: 12g
- Carbohydrates: 9g
- Fiber: 2g
- Sugar: 5g

Ingredient Substitutes:
- Experiment with different nuts and seeds like almonds or chia seeds.
- Swap dried cranberries for raisins or chopped dried apricots.
- Customize with a pinch of your favorite spice, such as nutmeg or cardamom.

CONCLUSION
A Culinary Symphony of Histamine Harmony

As you turn the last page of *"Low Histamine Cookbook,"* take a moment to savor the journey you've just embarked on. This isn't just a cookbook; it's a manifesto, a culinary rebellion against histamine havoc.

In these pages, you've discovered more than just recipes. You've uncovered a roadmap to a world where every ingredient is a choice, every preparation is a celebration, and every bite is a step toward a healthier, happier you.

Histamine intolerance may have thrown challenges your way, but you've emerged victorious with the help of Aveline's carefully curated meals. From detailed ingredients to foolproof methods, serving sizes that make sense, and nutritional empowerment, this book is your guide to rewriting the rules of your relationship with food.

But the journey doesn't end here. As you step into your kitchen, armed with this newfound knowledge, remember that each meal is an opportunity to embrace histamine harmony. Experiment, indulge, and savor the joy of eating without reservations.

Thank you for joining us on this amazing adventure. May your future meals be filled with not just sustenance but a symphony of tastes that harmonize with your body and soul.

Here's to Histamine Harmony – a revolution on your plate, and a celebration in every bite.

A HEARTFELT THANK YOU!

Thank you for your support on this culinary journey! If you enjoyed this book, please consider creating a video review or, if that's not feasible, leaving a written review. You can include a picture of the book or a page that caught your interest.

STEPS ON HOW TO LEAVE A REVIEW FOR THIS BOOK

1. Scan the QR code with your phone camera, a link will pop up on your screen, simply click on it to visit my author page.

2. Scroll down and locate the book titled "LOW HISTAMINE COOKBOOK " by Aveline Winter.

3. Once you find the book, click on its title to navigate to the book's sales page.

4. Scroll down on the sales page, and right after the "About the Author" section, you'll find the "Customer Reviews" section.

5. In the "Customer Reviews" section, you'll see an option to leave a review. Begin by rating the book with stars, indicating your overall satisfaction with it.

6. After rating, a text box or prompt will appear for you to leave a written review. Share your thoughts, experiences, and any feedback you have about the book.

7. Once you've written your review, double-check to ensure everything looks good, and then submit your review.

Your feedback is invaluable and greatly appreciated!
Thank you for taking the time to share your thoughts on
"LOW HISTAMINE COOKBOOK."

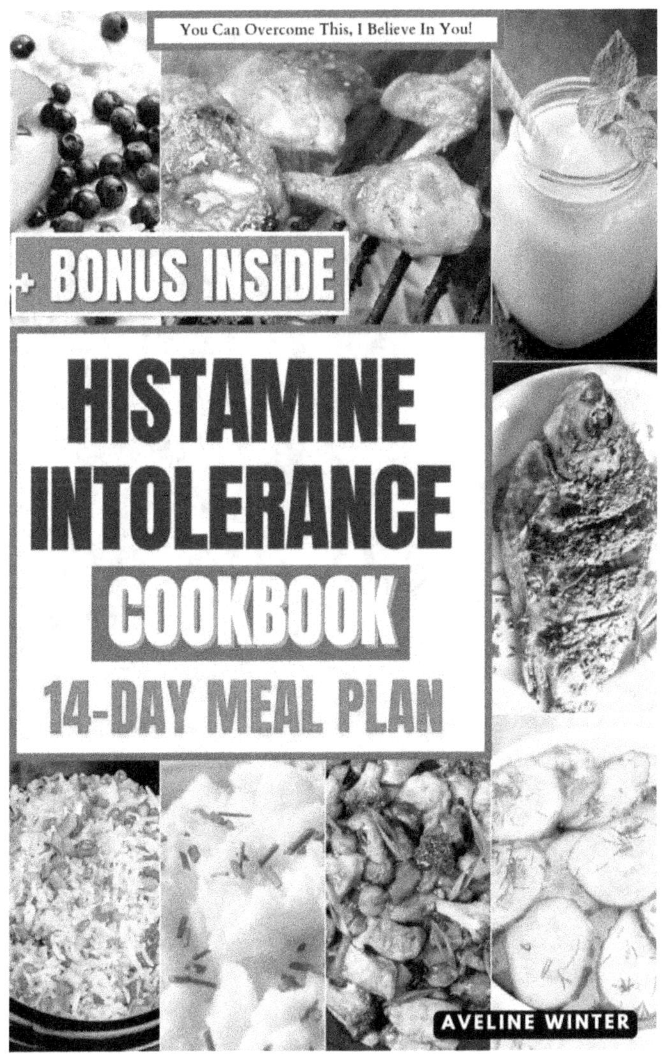
You Can Overcome This, I Believe In You!
+ BONUS INSIDE
HISTAMINE INTOLERANCE
COOKBOOK
14-DAY MEAL PLAN
AVELINE WINTER

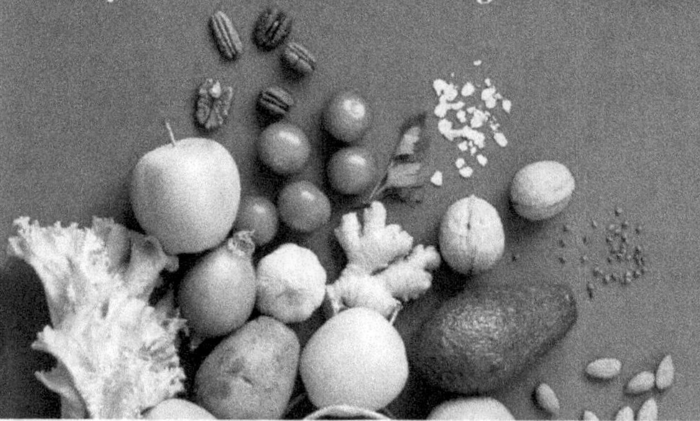

AVELINE WINTER
HISTAMINE
INTOLERANCE
FOOD LIST
The Complete Ingredient List - Your Guide to What to Eat, What to Avoid, and Why, Making Every Bite a Conscious and Delightful Choice.

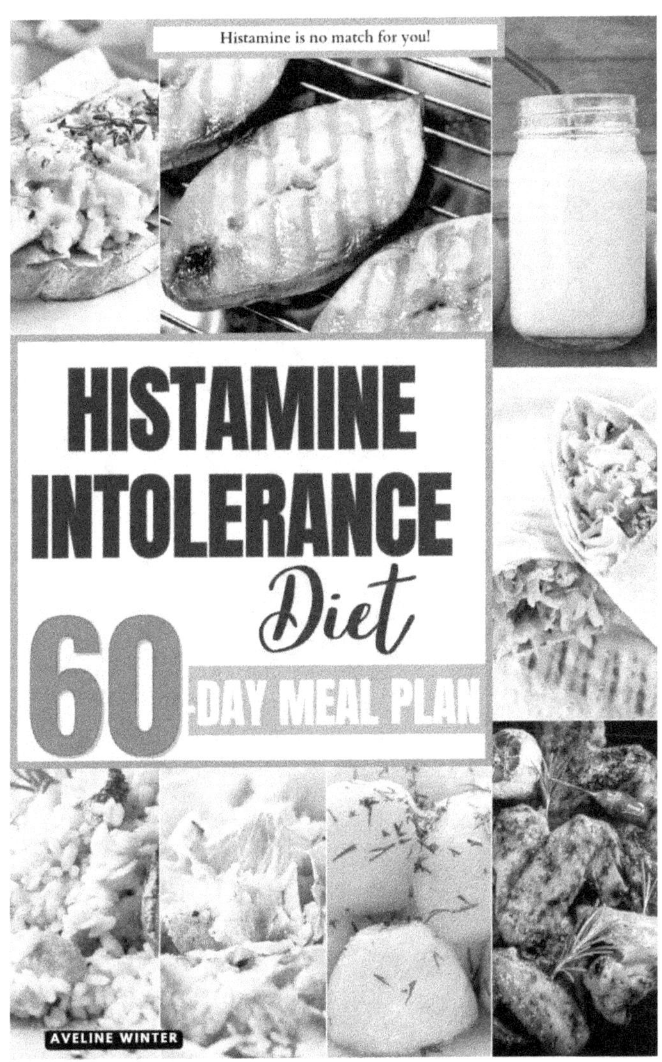

Histamine is no match for you!
HISTAMINE INTOLERANCE
Diet
60-DAY MEAL PLAN
AVELINE WINTER